Intermittent Fasting

A Comprehensive Guide To Shed Pounds, Boost
Metabolism, Lower Cholesterol, Improve Brain Health,
And Increase Energy Levels

I0135861

(Intermittent Fasting Improves Diabetes Management)

Rod-Andre Gravel

TABLE OF CONTENT

Introduction

Mary's wedding was in two months, and she was extremely anxious. She had always been a little on the plump side, but she had gained even more weight in the past year. She was unable to stop eating, and regardless of how much she exercised, she continued to gain weight.

She had heard that intermittent fasting could aid in rapid weight loss, but she was unsure if it would be effective for her. She decided to conduct research and discovered that many people had successfully lost weight through intermittent fasting.

She also discovered one of our articles that detailed everything she needed to know about intermittent fasting, including simple, nutritious, and delectable recipes to aid her on her journey. After reading the article, Mary determined that she wanted to try this. She was able to successfully incorporate intermittent fasting into her routine, and she experienced rapid results. She was able to lose the necessary weight for her wedding, and continued intermittent fasting afterward because she felt better than ever.

Following a vegan diet has also aided in my rapid and effortless weight loss, without the need to count calories or restrict my food choices. I've enjoyed being able to eat healthy, delicious meals while still fasting, and I've seen great results on my journey to lose weight. Moreover, the anti-inflammatory properties of a plant-based diet have helped alleviate my chronic joint pain. Switching to a vegan intermittent fasting lifestyle was one of the best choices I've made for my health and wellness.

My energy levels have increased, and my joint pain has diminished significantly. This change in lifestyle has made me happier and healthier, and I would highly recommend it to anyone seeking an effective weight loss strategy that also prioritises overall health and happiness.

Especially after the age of 40, when the metabolism begins to slow, intermittent fasting can be an effective weight loss method. This book explains the benefits of intermittent fasting and how to safely incorporate it into your weight loss programme. In addition, it includes 30 simple, nutritious, and delicious recipes that support intermittent fasting. In addition, there is a practical daily meal plan for rapid weight loss. This book will reveal the secrets of intermittent fasting and help you achieve your weight loss objectives.

Chapter 1: Why Should Women Practice Intermittent Fasting?

Intermittent fasting may seem like a good option for women who are interested in weight loss; however, a great deal of people wonder whether women should fast. Is intermittent fasting trustworthy for women? There have been a few important research studies on intermittent fasting, which can aid in weight loss for this intriguing new dietary trend.

Intermittent fasting is also referred to as alternate-day fasting, although there are variations on this diet. Recent research published in the American Journal of Clinical Nutrition involved 16 overweight men and women who participated in a 10-week programme. During the fasting days, individuals consumed only 25% of their estimated caloric needs. During the remaining time, they received dietary education; however, they were not given a specific criterion to adhere to.

This investigation was fascinating due to the fact that many individuals must lose even more weight than the researchers did before observing the same changes. It was a remarkable discovery that has inspired a large number of people to try fasting.

Intermittent fasting has beneficial effects for women. Women who adhere to a healthy diet and exercise regimen may have a problem with persistent fat. However, fasting is a reasonable remedy for this problem.

Intermittent Fasting for Women Beyond Menopause

During menopause, our bodies and metabolic rates change without question. One of the most significant changes that women over the age of 50 experience is a slowed metabolism that causes them to gain weight. Fasting is an excellent method for preventing weight gain and losing weight. Multiple research studies have demonstrated that this fasting pattern helps to control hunger. Additionally, those who adhere to it regularly do not experience the same desires as others. Suppose you are over the age of 50 and attempting to adapt to your slower metabolism. In this case, intermittent fasting can help you reduce your daily caloric intake.

At age 50, your body also begins to develop chronic conditions such as high cholesterol and high blood pressure. Even without a significant amount of weight loss, periodic fasting has been shown to decrease both cholesterol and blood pressure. Suppose you have begun to observe your numbers increasing annually at the doctor's office. In this case, you may be able to reduce them through fasting without losing a significant amount of weight.

Repetitive fasting may not be a good idea for every single woman. Anyone with a specific health condition or who frequently experiences hypoglycemia must consult a physician. This new dietary pattern has benefits for women, whose bodies naturally store more fat and who may have difficulty eliminating these fat deposits.

Chapter 2: Types Of Periodic Fasting

There are countless different ways to perform IF, which is astounding. If this is something you're interested in doing, you can find the approach that works best with your lifestyle, thereby increasing your chances of success. The following seven are listed:

This is among the most prevalent Whether strategies. The most distinguished book The FastDiet introduced it to the standard and explains everything you need to know about this method. The idea is to eat normally for five days (without counting calories) and then consume 500 or 600 calories per day, for women and men, on the remaining two days. The fasting days can be chosen according to personal preference.

The idea is that short periods of fasting keep you consistent; if you're feeling hungry on a fasting day, you should simply anticipate the next day, when you can "feast" once more. "Some people say, 'I can do anything for two days, but it's too much to restrict my diet every week,'" says Kumar. For these individuals, the 5:2 method may be more effective than calorie restriction throughout the week.

In general, the creators of The FastDiet advise against fasting on days when you plan to perform numerous endurance exercises. If you are preparing for a cycling or running race (or high-mileage weeks), consider whether this type of fasting is compatible with your training regimen. Alternatively, consult a sports nutritionist.

With this type of intermittent fasting, you choose a daily eating window that should ideally span a 14- to 16-hour fasting period. (Because of hormonal concerns, women should fast for approximately 14 hours each day.)

When liver glycogen is depleted, autophagy, the normal 'cell housekeeping' process in which the body eliminates waste and other substances that threaten the health of mitochondria, is accelerated by fasting. She says that doing so may aid in enhancing fat cell digestion and insulin capability.

Using this method, you might set your eating window from 9 a.m. to 5 p.m. Even so, it can serve a person with an early family dinner admirably. Consequently, a significant portion of the time spent fasting is energy spent resting regardless. (Depending on when you set your window, you do not actually need to "miss" any dinners.) Nonetheless, this depends on your dependability. If your schedule fluctuates frequently, or if you want or believe that you should have the opportunity to eat breakfast out irregularly, go out late at night, or attend parties, daily fasting may not be for you.

This method is the simplest of the package, and it consists of a daily 12-hour fast. For example: Choose to stop eating supper at 7 p.m. and then resume eating the following morning at 7 a.m. with breakfast. Autophagy does in fact occur at the 12-hour mark, but the cellular benefits are much milder. This is the minimum number of hours of fasting she recommends.

This strategy is simple to implement, which is one of its advantages. Similarly, there's no need to skip dinner; all you're doing is eliminating a bedtime snack (in the event that you ate one in the first place). This technique does not enhance the benefits of fasting in any way. If you're considering fasting for weight loss, a shorter fasting window means you'll have more opportunities to eat, and it may not help you reduce the number of calories you consume.

Stop Eating

This strategy was developed by Brad Pilon in his book Eat Stop Eat: The Incredible Truth That Makes Weight Loss Simple. Once more. His methodology differs from others in that he emphasises adaptability. Essentially, he emphasises that fasting is simply abstaining from food for a period of time. You engage in a few 24-hour diets per week and concentrate on an obstruction preparation programme.

"When your fast is complete, I believe you should pretend that it never occurred and eat normally. That is the end of the matter. Nothing more," he writes on his website.

Eating mindfully refers to returning to a normal approach to eating, where you don't binge because you just fasted, but also don't restrict yourself to an extreme diet or eat less than you want. Combining intermittent fasting with standard powerlifting is optimal for fat loss. By intermittently fasting for 24 hours during the week, you are able to consume slightly more calories on the other five or six non-fasting days. It makes it easier and more appealing to end the week with a calorie deficit without feeling as though you must adhere to an extreme diet.

This is a pick-your-own-experience approach to dealing with IF. You could perform time-restricted fasting (fast for 16 hours, eat for eight, for instance) every other day or more than once per week. This means that Sunday may be a typical day of eating, in which you stop eating at 8 p.m.; you would then resume eating on Monday around early afternoon. Essentially, it resembles skipping breakfast for several days or a week.

Something to remember: the research on the effect of skipping breakfast on weight loss is mixed. There is insufficient evidence to suggest that skipping breakfast affects weight. direct up bolt Nonetheless, a separate study demonstrates that eating breakfast can subtly influence weight loss. direct up bolt Another study has linked skipping breakfast with an increased risk of cardiovascular disease mortality. direct up bolt

This approach may be effectively adaptable to your lifestyle and is more about taking the path of least resistance, meaning you can make it work even if your schedule varies from one multiweek period to the next. However, a looser methodology may result in fewer benefits.

CHAPTER FOUR

Multivitamin, omega-3 supplement, rhobiotis, and vitamin D. As stated previously, I prefer whole foods to synthetic multivitamins. Therefore, I would use a greens supplement as my multivitamin. I obtain my omega-3 fatty acids from a high-quality fish oil or krill oil. For vegans, flaxseed oil or hemr oil would be an alternative. Regarding rheumatoid arthritis, the best source is naturally fermented foods like miso, kimchi, natto, kefir, and sauerkraut. Regarding urrlementation, choose one containing more than 10 billion astive rrobiotis train per serving. Vitamin D supplementation is vital for people who do not receive at least one hour of daily sun exposure. For example, if you live in the northeastern United States, you will need it. Because UV-B rays do not penetrate the skin as deeply as UV-A rays do, people with darker complexions will require more sun protection. Consequently, sunlight is converted into Vitamin D. Recent studies indicate that nearly everyone is deficient in vitamin D.

-

What is the finest Ture of Rrotein Rower to purchase?

It depends on your intended purpose. Whey is the most versatile protein. It absorbs fat, is crystalline, and is best taken after exercise. Casein rrotein is best taken before bed besause it is slowlu absorbed. I would recommend a protein powder made from grass-fed sow's milk due to its superior quality.

-Should I take my whey protein supplement before or after exercise?

Both, if you can afford it. The influx of branched-chain amino acids taken before your workout will enhance your performance. If you want to save money, you should take a protein supplement within 30 minutes of finishing your workout for recovery.

-

I Have Tried All Diets Without Success. How Can I Quickly See Results Without Dieting?

Intermittent fasting may be effective for you. Investigate why the 18th hour is the "golden hour." This is the time when you see the most results in the shortest amount of time. There are various theories regarding intermittent fasting.

Some say the fast begins immediately after our last meal, while others say it begins two or three hours later due to digestion. You should not sleep for more than 24 hours in a row. This is the point at which adverse effects on metabolism are observed, and honetlu, anything lasting longer than 24 hours is unbearable and distressing.

What foods are permitted during intermittent fasting?

Intermittent fasting involves not eating for a predetermined period of time. There are no interruptions during the meal course. That means that all foods are permitted. There are no temporary restrictions! And intermittent fasting does not limit the number or amount of calories consumed. Even consumers of junk food benefit from the daily meal break.

-

Are medications and nutritional supplements permitted during interval fasting?

During intermittent fasting, medications and dietary supplements can be taken as usual. Few supplements may be taken during lactation because they do not disturb the lactating rooster. Utilization of medication hould not be shanged on one's own volition, but only after consultation with a dostor.

Since intermittent fasting can reduce high blood pressure and increase insulin sensitivity, individuals taking medication for high blood pressure or high blood sugar should intermittently fast under close medical supervision. Here, if necessary, a dosage adjustment is required.

- Can alcohol be consumed during intermittent fasting?

Alcohol contains calories and is therefore prohibited during a fast. At the dining window, however, you may also order a beverage. Alcohol is not generally prohibited during intermittent fasting.

-

When is the optimal time to rort?

In principle, you can commit both fasting and food-related errors while intermittently fasting at the same time. There are no absolute rules present. If you want to burn fat effectively, you should train on an emrtu tomash because it stimulates fat metabolism and afterburn.

-

How long must I fast intermittently?

Intermittent fasting san be flexiblu designed. You san fast everu dau for 14, 16, 18, 20 hours or more. In the slais variant, 16-hour fasting periods alternate with 8-hour meal windows.

The optimal length of your meal break during intermittent fasting varies depending on your role. Again, there are distinctions that are unique to our profession.   neurotransmitter dominanse.

It is recommended that you begin with the slais variant, IF 16/8, and tau for four weeks. This is the best way to determine whether 16 hours of sleep per day is too much or too little for you.

-

Will I lose weight if I engage in intermittent fasting?

How much weight you lose through interval dieting depends on different factors. Your current weight, or how overweight you are, is just as important as the length of your meal break and, of course, what you consume during it.

There are numerous reports of people who have already lost weight using the IF 16/8 method without modifying their eating habits or caloric intake. On the other hand, there are reorle who must fast for at least 18 or 20 hours and/or pay close attention to their diet.

However, intermittent fasting is demonstrably superior to traditional dieting for weight loss. That's because insulin levels are low for an extended period of time due to intermittent fasting. This, in turn, is necessary for the body to convert stored fat into energy and maintain the basal metabolic rate. Consequently, you lose fat faster than muscle during interval fasting, and you need not worry about the infamous yo-yo effect that calorie-reduction diets induce.

-

How long should your interval be?

With intermittent fasting, you are not required to abstain from food permanently. There is no restriction. Favorite foods may still be consumed. This, coupled with the adaptable nature of the meal break, makes intermittent fasting extremely attractive for long-term use.

Intermittent fasting is neither a limited-time diet nor a passing fad. This is the "original life cycle" of man, in accordance with his biological design and the hormonal and neurobiological rhythms of the body.

Contrary to most diets, intermittent fasting is ideally suited as a permanent nutritional model. Short-term fating can prolong your life - and with a crystal-clear language!

-

Are exertions permitted while intermittently fasting?

It may occur that invitations, meetings, or other interruptions prevent you from taking your usual lunch break. Thankfully, this is not a broken leg. It was recommended that imrlu make an effort and consciously enjoy it, as opposed to being a social outsider with an angry appearance and a contentious argument.

Nor is it a tragedy when sixteen hours become fourteen or twelve hours. Perhaps you do not want to miss the weekend breakfast with your loved ones. All of this is without issue. Practicing IF 16/8 five or six days per week produces positive results.

However, it is recommended that you remain vigilant during the first day of the transition until you become accustomed to the meal breaks. Otherwise, there is a risk that you will not locate the IF-ruthm following the expression.

-Can I continue intermittent fasting if I'm sick?

If you are ill because you have a cold or the flu, it is best to listen to your body. If you are hungry, eat something, but do not neglect your responsibilities. When you are ill, you typically do not have an arretite anuwau. In our eue, this is a clear indication that the body does not require food, but rather channels all its energy into self-healing.

-Do I take enough nutrients with interval fasting?

Some individuals are concerned that they will not receive enough nutrients if they engage in interval fasting. However, intermittent fasting has a highly beneficial effect on the digestive tract. Long periods without food improve intestinal flora, allowing nutrients to be utilised more efficiently. There are no more effective measures to improve nutritional intake than daily meal breaks!

-

How frequently do you eat during mealtimes?

There is no rule dictating how frequently you should eat during interval fasting within your food window. So that everyone may handle it as they wish.

On the 16/8 interval fating method, individuals who consume small portions of food are still required to consume three meals per day. Other, on the other hand, do well with two large meals or a nask and a lavih main course.

Regardless of how you intend to implement intermittent fasting, you should allow at least three to four hours between meals from a physiological standpoint.

Chapter 3: How to Avoid the Drawbacks of the OMAD Diet

For some individuals, the OMAD diet may not be feasible.

Its major drawbacks include undereating, excess stress hormones, and possible reproductive problems. Patients with diabetes may also need to eat more frequently than the OMAD allows.

Undereating could be detrimental.

In one hour, it may be difficult to consume between 1,500 and 2,000 calories. Especially if you wish to adhere to a low-fat or vegetarian diet.

When nutrient-dense meat and healthy fats are used, OMAD becomes considerably more feasible.

If you are physically active or have a high caloric requirement, OMAD is likely not for you. It is simply too likely to lead to malnutrition. Nevertheless, it works for Herschel Walker, a former NFL player and MMA superstar.

Potential disadvantage: Stress Hormones

Changing to OMAD may induce hormonal changes in the body.

During the transition, your body may produce stress hormones like cortisol in order to mobilise protein for use as fuel.

Women may be more susceptible to cortisol-induced changes. If OMAD is too stressful for you, there are several other options for women's intermittent fasting.

Women who are pregnant or trying to conceive may want to delay OMAD use.

Intermittent fasting may result in hormonal imbalances and energy deficiency, which are risks that are not worth taking.

On the other hand, fasting does not appear to harm male fertility.

Chapter 4: Dietary Plans And Exercise Intermittent Fasting And The Keto Diet

Ketosis is the metabolic state in which the body uses ketones, which are derived from fat, rather than glucose, which is derived from carbohydrates. Fasting is characterised by ketosis, and ketogenic nutrition replicates the physiological effects of fasting.

If your diet is rich in carbohydrates, they will be converted to glucose and used to fuel your metabolism. If your diet is low in carbohydrates, below a certain threshold (20 g for most people, 30 or 50 g for some), your body will enter a state of ketosis, converting dietary lipids into ketones to use as an alternative fuel source.

As with alternative fuels for automobiles, this alternative fuel has many advantages: it is a fuel that is particularly suitable for specific organs, including the brain, which is why ketosis has therapeutic functions for people with neurological diseases such as epilepsy, Parkinson, and Alzheimer's, as well as for those suffering from migraines, depression, and... In addition, it is a "clean" fuel that produces minimal waste, such as free radicals. I can say that ketones have a unique anti-inflammatory effect on people with inflammation (pain, depression)

Fasting necessitates a state of ketosis in the body. In the absence of food, the body converts fat reserves into ketones and uses them as fuel.

Since the body does not expend energy during digestion, it can reserve this energy for other tasks, such as autophagy, or the process of cell recycling.

The ketogenic diet and fasting share similarities. I see fasting as an extreme form of the ketogenic diet as well.

To put the body into a state of ketosis, it is necessary to severely restrict carbohydrates by eliminating sugar and grains from the diet and replacing them with low-carbohydrate green vegetables, a small amount of animal protein (eggs, wild fatty fish, and grass-fed fatty meat), and appropriate lipids (coconut oil, olive oil, raw butter or ghee, duck fat, lard, avocado, olives, oil seed)

Dietary ketosis is an excellent aid for those wishing to fast. In fact, the body will adapt to the first few days of fasting more readily if it is already accustomed to using lipids as fuel. Also, after a few weeks, the ketogenic diet typically leads to a reduction in appetite, which again greatly facilitates fasting.

Therefore, a great way to prepare for fasting is to consume a ketogenic diet until the so-called keto-adaptation, which occurs when the body is able to carburize ketones. Once adaptation has occurred and hunger has subsided, adopt the intermittent fast by eliminating breakfast, followed by lunch or dinner, leaving only one meal per day. When the body is accustomed to eating only once per day, it is easily able to prepare for a longer fast. It is possible to fast without special preparation because, once in ketosis, the body will continue to rely on body fat for fuel in the absence of food and will not experience carbohydrate withdrawal symptoms. The day before a prolonged fast, a monodiète consisting of avocado, olives, or raw vegetables will aid in digestion.

Some people choose to drink only water or herbal teas during fasting. Vegetable or bone broths that have been filtered to contain only trace minerals and a small amount of salt can also be consumed for pleasure rather than nutrition. The purpose of fasting is to completely rest the digestive system. Peristalsis (the movement of food to the intestines) is completely halted, and the body can focus its energy on autolysis and autophagy, i.e., on eliminating excess fat and cells and cleansing the lymph and tissues. Additionally, hormones are balanced.

Pregnancy does not appear to be an appropriate time to begin a ketogenic diet or fasting. The future of young breastfeeding mothers will choose a low carb high fat (LCHF) diet, consisting of raw foods low in carbohydrates and rich in good fats, but a little more liberal than the strict ketogenic diet, i.e., they will keep some fruits or vegetables rich in starches, to adopt a Paleolithic diet, i.e., a diet similar to what our ancestors ate before agriculture. Some extremely rare individuals cannot adopt a ketogenic diet due to congenital deficiencies or metabolic disorders. Those who suffer from pulmonary tuberculosis or are on heavy medication should also avoid fasting.

The combination of intermittent fasting, long fasts, and ketogenic nutrition is especially effective for those who wish to lose weight and maintain their weight loss. Long-term, everyone will find his rhythm.

Chapter 5: How To Put Together Your Ketogenic Diet Program

One of the most difficult aspects of the ketogenic diet is preparing complete meals without grains, legumes, fruits, and vegetables that can disrupt ketosis, which ultimately promotes fat burning and weight loss.

Therefore, I will leave some suggestions for those who wish to implement this option in order to lose weight or gain muscle definition.

This plan should only be extended by 30 days, and you will observe your body gradually shedding those extra pounds. So that you can achieve your desired weight loss, it is crucial that you limit your consumption of hydrates and adhere to the guidelines of a healthy diet based on low-fat and nutrient-dense foods. In addition, it is highly recommended that you exercise regularly by going to the gym 3 to 5 days per week or playing sports in order to accelerate the burning of calories and the loss of accumulated fat.

TIPS FOR DOING THIS DIET

To be able to follow the ketogenic diet, you will need to modify some of your dietary guidelines and choose a much lower-calorie diet that will help you lose weight. To assist you in executing this plan, here are some suggestions:

PLAN YOUR MENU IN PHASES

I have already stated that this diet is divided into three phases, so it will be simple for you to grab a pen and paper and begin planning what you will eat each day of this phase. In this way, you will avoid the frustration of standing in front of the refrigerator unsure of what to eat, which can lead us to abandon this

38

diet. Therefore, the first step is to plan your meals and then go grocery shopping so that you only have consumable foods in your kitchen.

EMPTY YOUR PANTRY

To avoid succumbing to "temptations" during this method's 30-day duration, I recommend eliminating all caloric products that can attract your attention, such as cookies, muffins, pasta, etc. Give it to your family, your neighbour, or your friends to avoid having them at home and having to rummage through your closets in a fit of boredom or boredom.

TIME SPENT COOKING

To avoid becoming bored with the food you consume, it is best to be inventive with your recipes and explore new ways to eat healthily and lavishly. Consider that there are many ways to cook lightly, but that you will need to seek out information and, most importantly, invest a bit more time.

WEIGH YOURSELF ONCE A WEEK
It is one of the best ways to stay motivated and resist the temptation to abandon the diet. Therefore, create a ritual and weigh yourself completely naked once per week (at the same time) to determine how much weight you have lost; if possible, you should have a scale at home that not only displays your weight but also identifies your fat and muscle mass in order to evaluate the results of your efforts.

MENU OF THE FIRST PHASE OF THE KETOGENIC DIET
I am aware that the first phase of this diet is somewhat difficult to adhere to because not only are carbohydrates restricted, but many vegetables and fruits are also excluded. To determine

what to eat, it is best to assume that, during these days, you should primarily consume protein. I will provide an illustration to help you comprehend how to construct your diet:

• Breakfast: 1 cup of tea and 1 French omelette with skim cheese • Midmorning snack: 1 cup of skim yoghurt

• Lunch: Arugula salad with a tomato half and beefsteak

• Snack: skimmed yoghurt

• Dinner: lettuce salad with egg and tuna, plus one chicken drumstick baked in the oven

You should be aware that, by adhering to the guidelines of this diet, you will be able to lose between 1 and 3 kilogrammes per week (depending on your body composition and the excess kilogrammes) and up to 12 kilogrammes in one month!

Chapter 6: All About You Knew About Intermittent Fasting

We frequently engage in intermittent fasting without realising it, despite the fact that it sounds somewhat complex. When you eat, your body enters a state known as the "fed state," during which it absorbs and digests the food. Aside from when we sleep, many people remain in this "fed state" for the vast majority of the day.

Simply put, intermittent fasting refers to a period of time during which no food is consumed, typically between 12 and 48 hours. During this period, known as the "Fasting Window," only liquids such as water, herbal tea, and broth are permitted to be consumed.

Intermittent fasting is an age-old method for maintaining good health and general wellbeing. This potent healing technique has been used since the beginning of time, making it "ancient" and therefore "secret." However, we are learning about nutritional interventions because they have numerous benefits, including increased energy, weight loss, and reversal of type 2-9 diabetes, among others.

As there is no fixed duration for fasting, it is assumed whenever one is not eating. For instance, you fast between dinner and breakfast the following morning (approximately 12 to 14 hours).

The 5:2 Diet for Older Women

The 5:2 diet is based on the simple premise that you can eat whatever you want, including desserts, drinks, and pudding, five days per week. Then, women are restricted to 500 calories per day for two days per week that are not consecutive.

Professionals such as Professor Valter Longo, Professor in Gerontology and Biological Science at the USC, and Director of the Longevity Institute are conducting recent research in the United States. According to the source, calorie restriction may help you live longer, be healthier, improve your cognitive function, and lose weight.

There is still much human research to be conducted. I can guarantee that you will have a very positive experience with the 5:2 diet after the first year. Consult your physician before beginning the 5:2 diet. Before beginning any type of fast, those over the age of 60 who take medication or have health conditions such as diabetes or heart disease should consult a physician. There is still much human research to be conducted. I can guarantee that you will have a very positive experience with the 5:2 diet after the first year. Consult your physician before beginning the 5:2 diet. Before beginning any type of fast, those over the age of 60 who take medication or have health conditions such as diabetes or heart disease should consult a physician.

After receiving permission to fast, you should immediately purchase or download a calorie counter. Then download some low-calorie, nutritious recipes. Juices and smoothies do not need to be your sole source of nutrition throughout the day. When you don't have a lot of physical or social obligations, choose two days to fast. If you have never fasted before, begin gradually by extending the time between your last meal of the day and your first meal the following day.

If you eat at 7 p.m. and eat breakfast at 11 a.m. the next morning, you will have naturally broken a 16-hour fast. You determine when and how you consume your 500 daily calories. Experiment. Some individuals prefer to skip breakfast in favour of consuming all of their remaining calories at dinner, such as an egg on toast. Others are required to consume three meals per day, as well as low-calorie snacks such as crisp bread with low-calorie cream cheese and steamed vegetables in the evening, as well as large quantities of water and hot beverages.

Chapter 7: How Can I Fast?

Numerous individuals appreciate the fact that intermittent fasting offers a variety of options. You can practise intermittent fasting in a variety of ways, depending on your schedule and lifestyle. Some individuals fast on the few days per week when they are extremely busy. Some individuals enjoy restricting mealtimes and engaging in brief daily fasts.

You are free to choose the fasting method you employ. These strategies have the potential to be effective and deliver some of the desired benefits. Let's take a look at some of the available fasting options so you can choose the one that suits you best.

The 16/8 Method

This is one of the most popular methods for intermittent fasting. It entails eating during the remaining hours while fasting for approximately 14 to 16 hours per day. You may still consume two to three meals without consequence during this window. Although it still imposes restrictions so that you do not eat continuously throughout the day, it is more likely to be compatible with your typical eating schedule.

The procedure is easier than you might think. It is as simple as skipping breakfast or eating a late breakfast after your main meal. Thus, if your last meal is at 8:00 p.m. and you don't eat again until 12:00 p.m. the next day, you have fasted for 16 hours.

Breakfast could easily be served later in the morning. For example, if you had breakfast at 10 a.m. instead of 8 a.m. and finished eating by 6 p.m., you would still be within the 16-hour window. Some individuals have difficulty with this because they wake up hungry and believe they must consume breakfast.

This is the option you should select as an older woman.

14 to 15 hours between meals is more productive for women, so you should consider adopting this regimen.

During the fast, you may drink water, tea, coffee, and other non-caloric liquids to alleviate hunger pangs. Additionally, you must strive to consume only healthy foods during your eating window. During this time, it is not advised to consume a large amount of unhealthy foods. Some individuals adhere to a low-carb diet during an intermittent fast because it reduces hunger and improves results.

The 5:2 method

The 5:2 diet is an additional option available to you. In this plan, you are instructed to eat normally five days per week and consume no more than 600 calories on the other two. It is sometimes referred to as "the Fast diet."

On fasting days, it is recommended that men and women consume 600 calories each. For instance, although you would typically eat throughout the week, on Mondays and Thursdays you would only consume two modest meals with a total of 500–600 calories. As long as they are not consecutive, you may observe a fast on any day of the week. Select your two busiest days of the week and fast on those days.

The 5:2 diet has not yet been the subject of extensive research, but because it involves intermittent fasting, it is likely to produce the desired results.

You can complete tasks without worrying about food preparation throughout the day.

The Eat-Stop-Eat technique

On the Eat-Stop-Eat plan, you must fast for 24 hours once or twice per week. You can observe this fast while consuming one meal per day. The majority of individuals typically skip breakfast and lunch the day after dinner. This allows you to adhere to the 24-hour abstinence period without ever missing a meal.

During your fast, you may consume coffee, water, and other non-caloric liquids to stay hydrated, but no food is allowed. You are free to alter this as you see fit. If going from breakfast to breakfast or lunch to lunch is more convenient for you, you may select one of these options.

Keep in mind that you only fast one or two days per week. When it is time to eat regularly, you must consume the same amount of food as you would if you were not fasting. You may do so without endangering your health in order to lose weight.

The primary issue with this type of intermittent fasting is that it is difficult for the majority of people to fast for 24 hours. You may, however, ease into it. Before beginning a longer fast, you may find that beginning with a shorter fast, such as the 16-hour fast, can have some beneficial effects. It may be difficult to go an entire day without eating. Therefore, the majority of individuals choose one of the other fasting methods to achieve the same results.

Combat Diet

Regarding intermittent fasting, this is an additional popular option. The warrior diet encourages exercise and eating less during the day, when our ancestors were likely foraging for food instead of eating. The strategy is an adaptation of intermittent fasting that alternates periods of fasting with a brief window during which you can consume all the calories you need for the day.

The diet recommends quick workouts emphasising strength training, particularly for your back and joints, and fast-paced exercises like jumps, kicks, and sprints.

During the day, it is acceptable to consume raw fruits and vegetables, small amounts of protein, and liquids such as water, natural juices, coffee, and tea. Although many more recent iterations of the diet encourage undereating or fasting for twenty hours, the book specifies that this period should last between sixteen and eighteen hours.

Then you consume one substantial meal in the evening. There are no restrictions on the amount or type of food you can consume, so you are free to consume as much protein, fat, and carbohydrates as you desire.

Unplanned Meal Skipping

You can do this to prepare your body for intermittent fasting or to avoid worrying about when you will be able to eat. You'll sometimes miss some meals. During this fast, you do not need to worry about adhering to one of the more formal intermittent fasting strategies.

You may do this if you are not hungry or if you are too busy to eat. It is a common misconception that you must consume food every few hours to prevent starvation.

The human body is designed to endure extended periods of fasting. It is acceptable to skip a few meals, especially if you are not hungry or are extremely busy.

Theoretically, you are fasting whenever you skip two meals. If you are too busy to eat breakfast before leaving the house, ensure you have a nutritious lunch and supper. It is acceptable to skip a meal if you are running errands and cannot find a place to eat.

This will benefit you and save you time, so there is no harm done.

The results will likely not be as good as with other solutions, but it is still preferable to nothing and much easier to implement. Consider skipping one or two meals per week, or meals as needed. Clearly, if you are prepared to engage in intermittent fasting, you have a variety of options available to you. Some may be easier than others, and some may fit your schedule better than others. It is helpful to determine which fast you can most easily incorporate into your daily life.

Chapter 8: Does Intermittent Fasting Permit Any Type Of Beverage Consumption Without Breaking The Fast?

Intermittent fasting (IF) is a relatively new eating pattern that is frequently accompanied by high-protein or ketogenic diets. It is only natural to ask, "What is the optimal fasting plan?," "Will I experience negative side effects?" and "How much weight can I expect to lose?" Many individuals question whether they can consume beverages other than water and coffee while fasting.

Briefly, this diet is tailored to the consumption of beverages and the practise of intermittent fasting (IF) (various types of intermittent fasting, ranging from dry fasting to the Warrior

Diet, have different rules, abstain from consuming any calories during fasting.

Caution is advised against breaking the fast with any type of food, as this will negate the benefits of weight loss. Hypothesized benefits of intermittent fasting diets include decreased insulin resistance and improved blood sugar management, which may reduce the likelihood of developing diabetes. If you consume too much liquid during a fasting window, you will quickly lose the benefits.

It is important to know whether drinking any of the most commonly consumed beverages will break your fast if you are undergoing intermittent fasting.

Coffee

You may have it vertically. If you're attempting to lose weight, you can drink black coffee without ruining your diet. However, you should avoid sweetening or foaming the beverage with sugar, cream, or milk, as doing so can break your fast.

If you feel the need to add flavour to your coffee while fasting, try flavouring it with a spice such as cinnamon. Extra coffee should be consumed during nonfasting hours."

While adding fats to your coffee would technically be considered a violation of fasting principles, high-quality MCT is recommended for people who are consistently doing day-to-day intermittent fasting (IF) programmes, particularly if their goals are less about cutting calories and more about keeping blood glucose low and giving the body time to rest and digest.

When your objective is to increase your body's insulin sensitivity, fats do not have the same effect on blood glucose as carbohydrates or protein, so they will not hinder your fast. Due to the fact that the medium-chain lipids in MCT oil are immediately converted to ketones, an alternative fuel source for the brain compared to glucose, "many people report improved attention when drinking coffee with MCT oil in the morning."

If you must consume coffee during your fast, restrict yourself to one cup or switch to decaf. Consuming too much caffeine, especially on an empty stomach, may cause jitteriness and stimulate appetite.

Caffeine increases cortisol, which may cause you to feel anxious if you consume excessive amounts while fasting. Remember that cortisol is the stress hormone in the body.

Cortisol levels should be kept as low as possible during fasting to prevent the "cascade of hormonal responses" that can lead to elevated blood sugar. Extra caffeine consumption directly contradicts the purpose of fasting, which is to maintain low blood glucose and insulin levels.

Tea

Simply do it. As with coffee, it is acceptable to consume tea during a fast so long as it is prepared simply from tea bags, leaves, or flakes, with no added flavours or sweeteners. Choose unsweetened bottled iced tea to reduce calories and sugar content. Bottled iced tea is typically very sweet. When fasting, such beverages and foods containing extra calories, such as honey, milk, and cream, should be avoided.

Because tea naturally contains less caffeine than coffee, you can drink a bit more of it during a fast, but if possible, switch to decaf.

Seltzer and water

Because water is calorie-free, there is no need to restrict consumption. During fasts, drinking water is a good idea not only because it keeps you hydrated, but also because it helps you feel full and controls your appetite.

Adding fruit wedges or a true "splash" (approximately one tablespoon per 12 ounces) of lemon or lime juice (or a true "splash" of another juice) to water for flavour will add only a few calories. If carbonated water or seltzer is naturally flavoured and calorie-free, it can be used in the same manner as water.

Fermented apple cider vinegar

Unlikely to view it. Many people who fast believe that consuming ACV or an ACV tonic is safe. There are the same number of calories in apple cider vinegar and bone broth. Despite their diminutive size, consuming them would result in a metabolic break during a fast.

On the other hand, you're in luck if you enjoy drinking apple cider vinegar (ACV) or an ACV tonic even when you're not fasting. If your objective is to reduce daily calories, rest your digestive system, and reduce insulin levels, you have succeeded. However, apple cider vinegar is less likely than bone broth to increase insulin levels.

There are numerous intermittent fasting methods that may be suitable for different individuals. This diet adheres to basic guidelines.

A person must select and observe a 12-hour fasting window daily. According to some researchers, fasting for 10 to 16 hours can cause the body to convert its fat stores into energy and release ketones into the bloodstream. This facilitates weight loss.

This type of intermittent fasting plan may be suitable for beginners. This is due to the fact that the individual can consume the same number of calories each day, the fasting window is relatively brief, and the majority of the fasting occurs while the individual is asleep.

This is the most straightforward method, as it includes the time spent sleeping within the 12-hour fasting window.

A person could choose to fast from 7 p.m. to 7 a.m., if they ate dinner before 7 p.m. and breakfast at 7 a.m., but they would spend the majority of the time in between sleeping.

Chapter 9: The Manifestations Of Intermittent Fasting

The idea is that it is simpler to severely restrict caloric intake a few days per week or to limit eating to a smaller number of "eating periods" per day than to moderately restrict caloric intake at each and every meal, every day.

Proponents argue that fasting for longer durations (than the normal hour between meals) promotes cellular repair, improves insulin sensitivity, boosts the activity of human growth hormone, and modifies gene expression in ways that promote longevity and disease resistance. And what risks are there?

Before weighing the pros and cons of intermittent fasting, it is essential to understand that there are multiple types of intermittent fasting, and that there is insufficient evidence of their long-term safety and efficacy. The most prevalent varieties are listed below.

Intermittent fasting is also known as alternate day fasting.

Modified alternate-day fasting entails consuming only 25% of your normal caloric intake every other day.

Periodic fasting involves consuming between 500 and 600 calories per day on only two days per week.

Eating in a hurry, which restricts your daily "eating window"

Before deciding on an intermittent fasting plan that works for you, it is essential to discuss these potential side effects with a medical professional, as some plans may cause more symptoms than others.

Intermittent fasting may result in illness. Depending on how long they fast, people may suffer from headaches, lethargy, irritability, and constipation. To reduce some of these undesirable side effects, you may wish to switch from adf fasting to periodic fasting or a time-restricted eating plan that allows you to eat every day within a certain time frame.

It may result in overeating.

There is a strong genetic propensity to overeat following fasting periods, as your hunger hormones and brain's hunger centre ramp up when you are without food.

There is a risk of engaging in unhealthy eating habits on non-fasting days because it is human nature for people to want to benefit themselves after doing extremely difficult work, such as rigorous exercise or prolonged fasting.

According to a 2018 study, the two most common side effects of calorie-restricted diets — a slowed metabolism and an increased appetite — are just as likely to occur with intermittent fasting as with calorie restriction on a daily basis. And research on time-restricted eating is accumulating evidence that eating out of sync with a person's circadian rhythm is unhealthy.

In older adults, intermittent fasting may result in excessive weight loss.

Although intermittent fasting appears to have promise, even less is known about its benefits or how it may affect older adults. Human studies have concentrated on small groups of younger or middle-aged adults for brief durations. However, we are aware that intermittent fasting can be harmful in certain circumstances. If your body mass index is already marginal.

Certain medications may interact negatively with this substance.

Dieting and caloric restriction can be harmful for individuals with certain diseases, such as diabetes. Some individuals who take medications for hypertension or cardiovascular disease may be more susceptible to sodium, potassium, and other mineral imbalances during longer-than-usual fasting periods.

Chapter 10: Positive Aspects Of Intermittent Fasting

The primary benefits of intermittent fasting are weight loss and improved metabolic health, including better control of blood sugar in type 2 diabetes. Reduces Insulin Resistance, thereby enhancing blood sugar management.

Several studies have found that fasting improves blood sugar control, which may be particularly advantageous for diabetics. In fact, a study of ten people with type 2 diabetes found that intermittent fasting significantly reduced blood sugar levels.

Reduced insulin resistance can increase the body's sensitivity to insulin, allowing glucose to be transported from the bloodstream to the cells more efficiently. Combined with the possible blood sugar-lowering effects of fasting, this could help maintain stable blood sugar levels and prevent blood sugar spikes and crashes.

Improves Health by Combating Inflammation Acute inflammation is a normal immune response that aids in the fight against infections, whereas chronic inflammation can have severe consequences for health. According to research, inflammation may contribute to the development of chronic diseases such as cardiovascular disease, cancer, and rheumatoid arthritis. In addition to a small study, eight weeks of alternate-day fasting reduced blood triglyceride and "bad" LDL cholesterol levels by 25% and 32%, respectively (9Trusted Source). Another study involving 110 obese adults found that three weeks of fasting under close medical supervision significantly reduced blood pressure, blood triglyceride levels, total cholesterol, and "bad" LDL cholesterol.

Intermittent Fasting may enhance cognitive function and protect against neurodegenerative disorders: Numerous studies have found that fasting may have a significant effect on brain function. Since fasting may also reduce inflammation, it may help prevent neurological diseases. Non-age-related problems affecting the nervous system and the brain may be treated with fasting. Fasting improves brain function, prevents age-related cognitive decline, typically slows neurodegeneration, mitigates stroke-induced brain damage, and enhances functional recovery.

Reduces Calorie Intake and Increases Metabolism to Aid Weight Loss: Many dieters begin fasting in an effort to shed a few pounds rapidly and without difficulty. Theoretically, restricting your consumption of all or specific foods and beverages should reduce your total caloric intake, thereby accelerating your weight loss over time. In addition, a number of studies suggest that short-term fasting may increase metabolism by elevating norepinephrine levels, thereby facilitating weight loss. In addition, it was found that fasting protects muscle tissue more effectively than calorie restriction.

Intermittent Fasting stimulates the production of growth hormone, which is crucial for growth, metabolism, and muscle strength: Human growth hormone (HGH) is an essential protein hormone for many aspects of your health. In fact, studies indicate that this essential hormone influences muscle strength, growth, metabolism, and weight loss. Numerous studies indicate that fasting may increase HGH levels naturally. According to one study, a 24-hour fast significantly increased HGH levels in 11 healthy adults. Another small study involving nine men found that two days of fasting increased HGH production by a factor of five. In addition, some research suggests that sustained high insulin levels may decrease HGH levels, so fasting may help maintain constant blood sugar and insulin levels throughout the day.

Intermittent Fasting May Enhance Cancer Prevention and Chemotherapy Efficacy: A 2016 study found that the combination of fasting and chemotherapy decreased the spread of breast cancer and skin cancer. As a result of the combination of therapeutic strategies, the body produced more tumor-infiltrating lymphocytes and common lymphoid progenitor cells

(CLPs). CLPs derive from the white blood cells known as lymphocytes, which migrate into tumours and are known to destroy cancers. Short-term fasting increased stem cell production and made cancer cells more susceptible to treatment while sparing healthy cells, according to the same study.

Some studies have demonstrated that fasting reduces inflammation and promotes health: In a study published in Cell, Mount Sinai researchers discovered that fasting reduces inflammation and improves chronic inflammatory disorders without affecting the immune system's response to acute infections. Acute inflammation is a normal immunological mechanism that aids in the defence against pathogens, whereas chronic inflammation can have serious adverse health effects, such as heart disease, diabetes, cancer, multiple sclerosis, and inflammatory bowel diseases.

Reduces Blood Pressure, Triglycerides, and Cholesterol to Promote Heart Health: The leading cause of death worldwide, accounting for an estimated 31.5% of deaths, is heart disease (8Trusted Source). Dietary and lifestyle modifications are among the most effective ways to reduce the risk of heart disease. Some research suggests that incorporating fasting into your routine may be particularly beneficial for heart health.

Chapter 11: Why Does Intermittent Fasting Differ Between Men And Women?

Men and women respond differently to intermittent fasting. Women should be aware of possible threats to their overall health, bone health, and reproductive health.

Even if you are able to eat normally during non-fasting periods, certain forms of intermittent fasting may cause you to consume fewer calories. Your body obtains its energy from calories, and if there are insufficient calories, it will prioritise survival over other activities.

There is a paucity of research involving female participants, but rodent studies indicate that intermittent fasting may alter oestrogen levels and have a negative effect on reproductive processes such as menstrual regularity, fertility, pregnancy, and breastfeeding.

The disruption of male rats' hormone levels does not appear to have the same effect on their reproductive processes as it does on female mice. One possible explanation is that certain aspects of female reproduction, such as pregnancy and lactation, require more energy than their male counterparts.

Consequently, inadequate energy intake may have a negative effect on these processes. It is currently unknown whether female humans are affected similarly to female rodents.

A growing body of evidence suggests that calorie restriction may also weaken bones and reduce bone density.

However, compared to calorie-restricted diets, intermittent fasting does not appear to have the same impact on bone mineral density.

To address these health risks, women may need to approach intermittent fasting differently than men do. It may be possible to reduce adverse side effects by implementing gradual, moderate changes over time as opposed to drastic ones. Consult your physician if you are considering intermittent fasting to learn about any potential risks and to determine if it is appropriate for you.

We've discovered that everyone reacts differently to food. The fact that even identical twins react differently to the same meal suggests that our metabolic health is neither inherited nor fixed.
With the at-home test, you can determine which of the 15 "good" and 15 "bad" gut bugs we've identified reside in your stomach. These are associated

with an increased or decreased risk of type 2 diabetes, cardiovascular disease, and abdominal fat.

The test evaluates your blood sugar and blood fat responses to food, as well as your gut bacteria, and uses the most recent research to determine which foods are optimal for your metabolism.

Chapter 12: What Are The Finest Foods To Consume Throughout A Non-Fasting Window?

During intermittent fasting, it is essential to prepare a balanced meal in order to maintain optimal health. During periods of fasting, it is essential to choose nutritious meals to meet daily nutritional needs. You must focus more on consuming protein-rich meals, low-carb whole grain foods, and healthy fats. This post will discuss what to eat after fasting.

Surely, water is not food. But it is a crucial factor that will aid you in intermittent fasting. During a 16-hour fast, the body metabolises the glycogen-bound sugar stored in the liver. During fasting, your body expends energy and consumes electrolytes. Therefore, it is essential to stay hydrated.

However, the amount of water you should consume depends on factors such as your age, gender, and weight. Experts recommend that adults consume at least eight glasses of water per day. Water consumption increases blood flow and prevents dehydration. Dehydration poses a risk for a variety of health conditions, including fatigue, nausea, weight gain, and lethargy.

The colour of your urine is an excellent indicator of your dehydration. Urine should generally be pale yellow; if it is dark yellow, it indicates that your body is becoming dehydrated.

Some of the best foods for intermittent fasting include vegetables such as broccoli, cabbage, cauliflower, and brussels sprouts. They are composed of fibre. In order to prevent constipation, it is essential that you consume additional fibre between meals.

Cruciferous vegetables are abundant in vitamins C, E, and K, as well as beta-carotene, minerals, and antioxidant activity. Numerous studies indicate that the antioxidant properties of these vegetables fight cancer. They make you feel full, allowing you to fast for a longer duration.

Avocado is a nutrient-dense, whole food that prevents weight gain and reduces the risk of obesity. Avocados are low-calorie fruits that help prevent obesity.

Avocados' dietary fibre reduces weight gain by increasing satiety and preventing fat absorption.

Mannoheptulose is a weight loss-promoting monosaccharide. Avocado is rich in MUFAs, which prevent fat accumulation and aid in the elimination of excess fat. After a period of fasting, it is necessary to consume healthy fats.

There is evidence that avocados promote satiety and reduce appetite and food consumption. Avocado also alters gut hormones; this would eventually benefit calorie consumption and weight management.

SEAFOOD
According to the Dietary Guidelines for Americans, each week you should consume at least two to three ounces of

fish. Fish, shrimp, and other seafood are rich in protein, vitamin D, and healthy fats.

Seafood is an excellent option for a fasting meal because it is nutrient-dense and does not add extra calories to your diet.

Fish consumption is heart-healthy and reduces cardiovascular risk. Fish is strongly recommended as part of an intermittent fasting diet.

Carbohydrate-rich foods provide energy for daily activities; therefore, it is essential to include some low-calorie carbs in your diet. Legumes and beans are low-calorie, protein- and mineral-rich carbohydrates.

Legumes and beans aid in satiety during the hours of fasting. Beans, peas, lentils, and chickpeas are associated with weight loss, even in the absence of calorie restriction.

EGGS

The eggs are protein-rich and can be produced in mere minutes. It is recommended to include eggs in your intermittent diet, as they help you feel full and provide the necessary nutrients.

White potatoes can be quickly absorbed and are an excellent addition to your intermittent fasting meal plan. It is a fantastic post-exercise snack when combined with a protein source. It may replenish your muscles' energy. Potato starch is beneficial for intestinal microbes.

FRUITS AND BERRIES

Fruits and berries are rich in vitamins, minerals, and carotenoids, making them healthy and nutritious. We recommend consuming a bowl of mixed fruits and berries. These fruits promote satiety and good health. The recommended daily intake of fruits and vegetables is 400 grammes.

Fruits aid in the breakdown of proteins and facilitate digestion. In addition, they result in improved skin health, less cell damage, and weight loss.

You may include a variety of nuts in your diet because they contain excellent fats. They are excellent alternatives for satisfying hunger during intermittent fasting. Nut consumption lowers the risk of cardiovascular disease, type 2 diabetes, and death.

WHOLE GRAINS

Whole grains are high in dietary fibre, so they can help you feel full and manage your weight. Wheat, whole wheat bread, pasta, oats, millets, buckwheat, brown rice, and cracked wheat are examples of whole grains.

Whole grains have been linked to a reduced risk of cardiovascular disease, diabetes, and certain cancers, among other health issues.

GHEE

Ghee is abundant in omega-3 (DHA) and omega-6 (CLA) fats, which are beneficial for weight loss. The short-chain fatty acids in ghee assist in accelerating the digestive process.

Omega 6 fatty acids have been linked to an increase in lean body mass and a reduction in fat mass. It also helps mobilise fat cells for energy production.

PROBIOTICS
It is recommended to consume a probiotic beverage while intermittent fasting. It supports gut flora and promotes better digestion.

Probiotics assist in regulating the number of beneficial bacteria in the gastrointestinal tract and reducing the symptoms of irritable bowel syndrome.

Additionally, intermittent fasting with probiotics improves glucose tolerance and helps prediabetics achieve weight loss and glycemic improvement.

SMOOTHIES

Smoothies made with peanut butter, avocado, berries, bananas, and dry fruits can help you meet your nutritional requirements. Smoothies that are nutritious and healthy may help you feel full. They provide an abundance of vitamins, minerals, and proteins.

You may also include sugar-free fresh fruit juice in your diet; it aids in weight loss and is rich in nutrients. Remember that juice should be consumed throughout your mealtime. During fasting, only non-caloric beverages such as water, black coffee, and plain tea are permitted.

Chapter 13: Intermittent Fasting

Intermittent fasting is a diet plan that alternates between brief fasting intervals in which the dieter consumes no or significantly fewer calories than usual. Intermittent fasting is designed to increase the length of time your body is in a fasted state.

It is marketed to alter body composition via weight loss and a reduction in body fat, and to improve disease-related health indicators such as blood pressure and cholesterol levels. Its roots lie in traditional fasting, a worldwide practise documented in the earliest writings by Socrates, Plato, and religious organisations as having physiological or spiritual benefits.

The objective of intermittent fasting is to drastically reduce caloric intake for brief periods, as opposed to deprivation.

It is believed that eating smaller portions can satisfy the body and reduce cravings for unhealthy snacks. As long as you continue to eat healthily while experimenting with everything, you can try everything.

What is the function of intermittent fasting?

Although intermittent fasting can be performed in a variety of ways, all begin with the selection of a regular eating schedule and a fasting period. You could, for instance, try fasting for the remaining sixteen hours of the day and eating only eight hours per day. Or, you could choose to skip two meals per week and consume only one meal per day. To comprehend how intermittent fasting promotes fat loss, one must first comprehend the distinction between the fed and fasted states.

The fed state occurs when your body is actively absorbing and digesting food. The fed state typically lasts between three and five hours as the body assimilates and digests the food that was just consumed.
In a fed state, insulin levels are quite elevated, making it very difficult for the body to metabolise fat.

After that, the body enters the post-absorptive period, which is a fancy way of saying that it is no longer digesting food. Until 8 to 12 hours after your last meal, you are in the post-absorptive state; then, you enter the fasted state. Your body burns fat significantly more efficiently during a fast because insulin levels drop. When you are fasting, your body can access fat reserves that were unavailable when you were fed.

Our bodies rarely experience this fat-burning stage because we don't enter the fasted state until 12 hours after our last meal. This is one of the reasons why many individuals who begin intermittent fasting experience fat loss without altering their diet, caloric intake, or level of physical activity. When you fast, your body enters a mode of fat-burning that is unusual during a normal eating schedule.

Intermittent fasting (IF) can be effective in two ways: caloric restriction (consuming fewer calories than needed) and reduced meal frequency (number of meals/snacks consumed daily).

Salad of avocado and fennel dressed with balsamic vinegar

- 1 cup mandarin oranges, drained
- 2 cup chopped romaine lettuce
- ½ teaspoon freshly ground black pepper
- 2 tablespoon light olive oil
- one tablespoon of balsamic vinegar
- ½ teaspoon salt
- 1 cup fennel, sliced
- 1 avocado, diced

Whisk together the olive oil, balsamic vinegar, salt, and pepper in a medium mixing bowl until well combined and slightly thickened.

This is your balsamic dressing.

Add the fennel, avocado, oranges, and lettuce to the dressing and toss until the vegetables are evenly coated.

Serve cold, divided between two salad plates.

Flavorful Chocolate Keto Fat Bombs

2 tablespoon ground cinnamon
½ teaspoon kosher salt
1 cup toasted coconut flakes
½ teaspoon cayenne (to taste)
¼ cup coconut oil
¼ cup smooth peanut butter
1 cup dark cocoa
5 (6 g) packets of stevia (or to taste)

DIRECTIONS

In a double boiler set above a pot of boiling water, combine peanut butter, coconut powder, and cocoa powder.

Stirring it frequently, heat it until melted and smooth, whisking it frequently.
Stir together the stevia, cinnamon, and salt until thoroughly combined.
Fill a silicone mini muffin pan with the mixture halfway.

Summary

Surely you've heard of success stories involving intermittent fasting and muscle growth and fat loss. This is not a fad diet, but rather a shift in your eating habits that is effective. The claims that it is possible to lose weight while maintaining or gaining muscle are entirely accurate, as I have personally experienced this phenomenon.

By following this plan, you can anticipate losing at least two pounds per week. If you're doing everything correctly, you should have no trouble obtaining this sum. The aforementioned intermittent fasting exercise routine is designed to help you gain muscle mass while losing weight.

Without a doubt, you may lose more than two pounds per week if you adhere to this diet. If you are extremely overweight, this is acceptable, but if you are slightly overweight, you must slow down. In general, it is optimal to lose no more than two pounds per week.

Final Remarks
Combining fasting and exercise is one of the most effective methods for losing weight rapidly. Intermittent fasting is a pattern of eating that helps create a caloric deficit, just as exercise burns calories. If you struggle to lose weight or need to lose weight quickly, you may find the above workout to be extremely beneficial.

Fasting and exercise are particularly effective if you are attempting to get extremely lean or if you are extremely overweight to begin with. When you are thin, with 8-10% body fat, it becomes difficult to continue losing weight because your body begins to retain essential fat. It is easier to achieve the calorie deficit required to become even slimmer if you are not eating.

Finally, nothing on this page should be construed as medical advice. Intermittent fasting is a successful method of weight loss for many people, but that does not mean it will work for you. Before adopting a new eating pattern, you should conduct a comprehensive study and make lifestyle changes at your own risk. Consult your physician or a registered dietitian if you have any questions or concerns.

Conclusion

Intermittent fasting is the practice of going without food for periods that are both regular and brief. Numerous studies have been conducted on intermittent fasting, and they all highlight the benefits of this eating pattern. Intermittent fasting is a pattern of eating that can and must be adapted to fit anyone's lifestyle and level of expertise, regardless of the number of different approaches that have been developed for it. This is the most important aspect of this type of diet to comprehend. You may feel better if you follow a modified version of the 16:8 (such as a 10:14, 12:12, etc.) or if you go two days without eating, to name a few possibilities. It is also possible that you will discover that fasting has no effect on your body!

Use intermittent fasting to learn about yourself, your body, and your mind: Despite the fact that weight loss is one of the most common reasons why people adopt the intermittent fasting (IF) pattern, this routine is advantageous in so many ways that it is difficult to abandon. Find a rhythm, pattern, or routine that makes you feel good and use intermittent fasting to learn about your body.

Regarding food, health, and nutrition, there is no universally applicable silver bullet solution. The diet that works best for you is one that you can maintain over time by adapting it to your lifestyle and nutritional needs.

www.ingramcontent.com/pod-product-compliance
Lightning Source LLC
Chambersburg PA
CBHW070525030426
42337CB00016B/2106